Natural Solution to Eye Problems

The Care for Eye Vision

Deirah Jelloy

Copyright © 2020 by Deirah Jelloy

All rights reserved. No part of this publication may be reproduced, distributed, or transmitted in any form or by any means, including photocopying, recording, or other electronic or mechanical methods, without the prior written permission of the publisher, except in the case of brief quotations embodied in critical reviews and certain other non-commercial uses permitted by copyright law.

ISBN: 978-1-63750-204-4

Table of Contents

NATURAL SOLUTION TO EYE PROBLEMS 1

INTRODUCTION 5

CHAPTER 1 7
    STRUCTURE OF THE EYE 7

CHAPTER 2 10
    EYE PAIN: WHAT ARE THE CAUSES? 10
    COMMON EYESIGHT PROBLEMS 11
    ASSESSMENTS TO DIAGNOSE EYES PAIN 15
        Treatments *15*

CHAPTER 3 18
    TOP FACTORS BEHIND EYE PROBLEMS 18

CHAPTER 4 32
    INFECTIONS OF THE EYE 32
    SYMPTOMS OF THE EYE INFECTION 33
    TYPES OF VISION INFECTIONS 34
        How come there gunk in my eye? *36*

CHAPTER 5 39
    VISION FLOATERS: CAUSES, SYMPTOMS, AND TREATMENT 39
    WHAT ARE THE SYMPTOMS? 39
    WHAT CAUSES THEM? 40
        How Are Floaters Treated? *43*

CHAPTER 6 45
    WHAT ARE EYE FRECKLES? 45
    WHAT CAUSES EYE FRECKLES? 47
    DO EYES FRECKLES NEED TREATMENT? 47

CHAPTER 7 50

Eye Twitch 50
What are the Types of Twitches? 52
How could it be Treated? 54

CHAPTER 8 57

Red Spot of the Eye 57
How are they Diagnosed? 59
How Are They Treated? *59*

CHAPTER 9 61

Diabetes and Eye Problems 61
Cataracts 62
Glaucoma 62
Treatment *63*
Prevention - Have your eyes doctor display for glaucoma annually. *63*
Retinopathy 64
Treatment *64*

CHAPTER 10 66

Glossary of Eye Terms 66

Introduction

This book is aimed at providing natural solution to eye problems. In this book; you would learn the fundamental causes of eye problems, eye infections and its symptoms and subsequently its treatment.

The eye is an organ that reacts to light and allows vision; the cells in the retina that allows mindful light belief are, which also enables eyesight, including color differentiation and the understanding of depth.

Also; you would learn the top factors that contribute to eye problems, such as red spot of the eye, eye twitch, vision problems and diabetes, cataracts, glaucomaretinopathy and freckles. You would likewise learn more about vision terms.

After reading this book, I believe you would be glad you have read.

The eye can differentiate between about 10 million colors and has the capacity to detect an individual photon.

Like the eye of other mammals, the human being eyes

non-image-forming photosensitive ganglion cells in the retina receive light indicators which affect modification of how big is the pupil, regulation, and suppression of the hormone melatonin and entrainment of your body clock.

Chapter 1

Structure of The Eye

Blood vessels are seen within the sclera, and a strong limbal band round the iris.

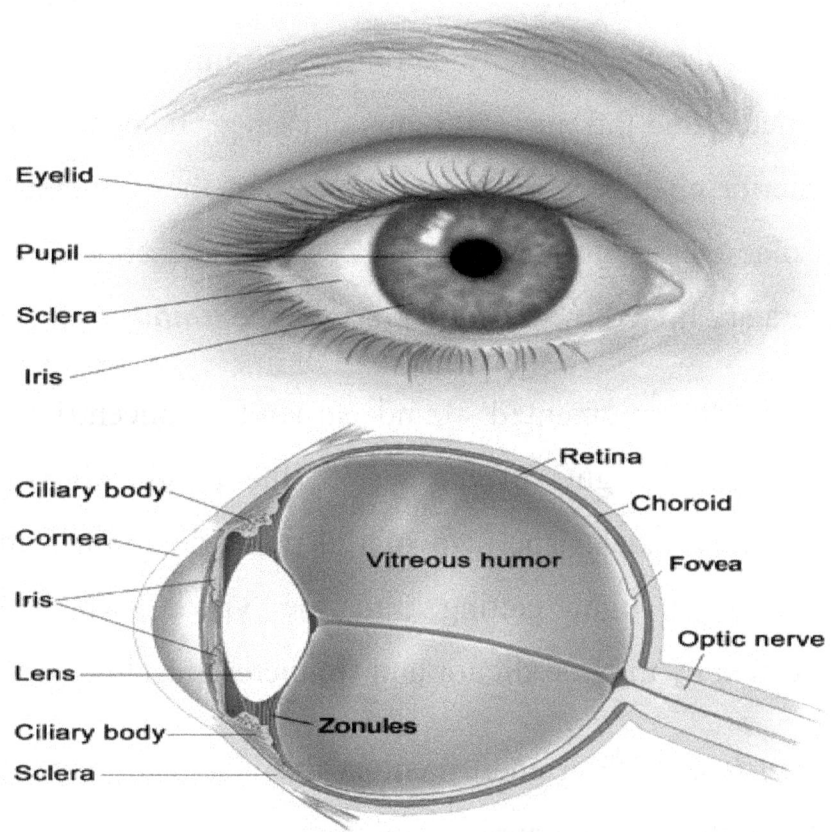

The outer elements of the eye:

The vision is made up of the anterior segment and the

posterior segment; it's not shaped just like a perfect sphere. The anterior section comprises of the **cornea, iris, and zoom lens.**

The cornea is clear and more curved, and it is from the bigger posterior portion, made up of the *vitreous, retina, choroid, and the external white shell called the sclera.* The cornea is normally about 11.5 mm (0.3 in) in diameter, and 0.5 mm (500 μm) thick near its center, the posterior chamber constitutes the rest of the five-sixths; its diameter is normally about 24 mm. The cornea and sclera are linked by a location termed the **limbus.**

Iris is the pigmented round structure concentrically encircling the guts of the vision, the pupil, which is apparently black. The size of the pupil determines the quantity of light getting into the vision, which is modified by the iris' dilator and sphincter muscles.

Zoom lens - Light energy enters the vision through the cornea, through the pupil and then through the zoom lens; the lens form is transformed for near focus (accommodation), and it is managed by the ciliary muscle. Photons of light dropping on the light-sensitive cells of the retina (photoreceptor cones and rods) are changed into electric indicators that are sent to the mind by the optic nerve and interpreted as view and vision.

Chapter 2

Eye Pain: What are the causes?

Nearly everyone will establish sore eyes sooner or later; sometimes, they progress independently, but they may also be an indicator of something much more serious. Your eye doctor can find out what's happening and discover the right treatment for you.

Where will it hurt?

Sometimes pain results from a problem in your eyesight or the parts around it, such as:

- <u>Cornea</u>: The clear windows in leading of your eyes that concentrate light.

- <u>Sclera</u>: The whites of your eyes.

- <u>Conjunctiva</u>: The ultra-thin covering of your sclera and the within of your eyelid.

- <u>Iris</u>: The colored part of your vision, with the pupil in the center.

- Orbit: A bony cave (vision socket) in your skull where the eye and its muscles can be found.

- Extraocular muscles: They rotate your eyesight.

- Nerves: They carry visual information from your eye to the human brain.

- Eyelids: Outdoors coverings that protect and pass on dampness over your eye.

Common Eyesight Problems

- Blepharitis: An swelling or infections of the eyelid which typically is not painful

- Conjunctivitis (pinkeye): That is irritation of the conjunctiva. It could be from allergy symptoms or attacks (viral or bacterial). Arteries in the conjunctiva swell. It makes the part of your eyes that's usually white look red. Your vision may possibly also get itchy and gunky. This problem usually is not painful.

- Corneal abrasions: That's the state name for a

scratch upon this part of your vision. It sounds minimal, but it can harm. It's easy to do, too. You are able to scratch your eyesight while massaging it. Your physician will provide you with antibiotic drops. It will progress in a few days without further problems.

- <u>Corneal infections (keratitis)</u>: A swollen or contaminated cornea may also be the effect of a bacterial or viral infection. You might be much more likely to obtain it if you leave your connections in overnight or wear filthy lenses.

- <u>International bodies</u>: Something in your eye, like a little of dirt and grime, can irritate it. Make an effort to wash it out with artificial tears or drinking water. If you don't obtain it out, it can scrape your eye.

- <u>Glaucoma</u>: This category of conditions causes liquid to develop in your eyes, which places pressure on your optic nerve. If you don't address it, you could lose your view. More often than not, there are no early symptoms. But a sort called severe angle-closure glaucoma; causes pressure within your vision to rise all of a sudden. Medical indications include severe vision pain, nausea and throwing up, headaches, and worsening eyesight. It is an urgent situation. You will need treatment ASAP to avoid blindness.

- <u>Uveitis</u>: A swelling inside your eyesight from trauma, attacks, or issues with your disease fighting capability. Medical indications include pain, red eyes, and, often, worse eyesight.

- <u>Optic neuritis</u>: An inflammation of the nerve that travels from the trunk of the eyeball into the human brain. Multiple sclerosis and other conditions or attacks are often at fault. Symptoms include lack of eyesight and sometimes deep distress when you look laterally.

- <u>Sinusitis</u>: Contamination in another of your sinuses. When pressure accumulates behind your eye, it can distress using one or both edges.

- <u>Stye</u>: That is a sensitive bump on the advantage of your eyelid; it happens when an essential oil gland, eyelash, or locks follicle gets contaminated or inflamed. You might hear your physician call it a *chalazion or hordeolum.*

Other Symptoms

Eye pain can occur alone or with other symptoms, like:

- Less vision.

- Discharge (It could be clear or solid and colored)

- Foreign body sensation (the sensation that something is in the vision, whether real or imagined)

- Headache.

- Light sensitivity.

- Nausea/vomiting.

- Red-eye or pinkeye.

- Tearing

Your eye is crusted shut with discharge when you awaken. Other symptoms, along with a sore eye, can be considered a clue from what is leading to the pain.

Assessments to Diagnose Eyes Pain

See your eyes general practitioner if you have eye pain, particularly if you have less vision, headache, or nausea and throwing up.

Vision doctors use some tools to diagnose vision pain:

- A slit-lamp exam uses shiny light to check out all the constructions of your vision.

- Dilating drops increase your pupil to allow doctor to see deep into the eye.

- A tonometer is an instrument that measures eyesight pressure. The physician uses it to diagnose glaucoma.

Treatments

Just like causes may differ, so do treatments. They focus on the specific reason behind eye pain.

- *Conjunctivitis*: Antibacterial eye drop could cure bacterial conjunctivitis. Antihistamines by means of eyes drop, a tablet or syrup can improve conjunctivitis from allergy symptoms.

- *Corneal abrasions*: These heal independently with time. Your physician might recommend an antibiotic ointment or drops.

- *Glaucoma*: You'll get eyes drop and perhaps pills to lessen pressure. If indeed, they don't work, you might need surgery.

- *Infected cornea*: You might need antiviral or antibacterial eye drop.

- *Iritis*: The physician will regard this with steroid, antibiotic, or antiviral eyes drop.

- *Optic neuritis*: It's treated with corticosteroids.

- *Styes*: Use warm compresses at home for a couple of days.

The only path to straighten out the sources of eye pain

and also to get the right treatment is to see a medical expert. Your eyesight is valuable; protect it by firmly taking eye pain significantly.

Chapter 3

Top Factors behind Eye Problems

A lot of people have eyesight problems at one time or another. Some are small and will disappear independently (easy to take care of at home), while others need a specialist's treatment. Whether your eyesight isn't what it used to be, or never was that great, there are actions you can take to get your eyes health back on the right track.

Below are some common sight problems;

- **<u>Eyestrain</u>**

Anyone who reads all night, works with a pc, or drives long distances is vulnerable to this problem; it happens when you overuse your eye, they get exhausted and need to rest, exactly like some other part of the body.

In case your eyes feel strained, provide them with a while off. If they're still weary after a couple of days, consult with your doctor to ensure it isn't another problem.

- **Red-Eyes**

Your eyes look bloodshot. Why?

This is when the surface of the eye is protected in arteries that expand when one is annoyed or infected, which causes the red look.

Red-eye is actually a symptom of another eye condition, like conjunctivitis (pinkeye) or sun damage from not sporting shades over time. If over-the-counter vision drops and rest don't clear it up, see your physician.

Eyestrain can be the solution to this problem, therefore just a little sleep at night is enough. If a personal injury is the reason, get it examined by your physician.

- **Night Blindness**

This is a sight problem that makes it difficult for one to see at night, stay on course around any dark places. *Nearsightedness, cataracts, keratoconus, and too little supplement A; all result in a type of evening blindness that doctors can fix.*

Some individuals are born with this issue, or it could

develop from a degenerative disease relating to the retina, and that always can't be treated. *When you have it, you'll have to be extra careful in regions of low light.*

- **Lazy Eye**

Sluggish eye, or amblyopia, happens when one eye doesn't develop properly; this happens when "the particular eye" vision is weak, and it will move "lazily" around as the other eye remains put. It has been observed to happen mostly amidst babies, children, and adults, and hardly ever affects both eyes.

Treatment must be sought immediately for newborns and children; lifelong vision problems can be prevented if a sluggish eye is recognized and treated during early childhood. *Treatment includes corrective contacts or glasses and utilizing a patch or other ways of making a kid use the sluggish eye.*

- **Cross Eye (Strabismus) and Nystagmus**

In case your eyes are not prearranged with one another when you take a look at something, you might have *strabismus*; this is also known as crossed eye or walleye. This issue won't disappear completely unless you get an ophthalmologist, or eyes specialist, to improve it.

There are numerous treatments, including vision therapy, to make your eyes stronger. Surgery is also a choice. Your physician will test your eye to see which treatment might work right for you.

- **Colorblindness**

When you can't see certain colors, or can't tell the difference between them (usually reds and greens), you might be colorblind; it happens when the color cells in your vision (the physician will call them cone cells) are absent or don't work.

When it's most unfortunate, you can only just see in tones of gray, but this is rare. A lot of people who've it are given birth to with it; nevertheless, you can obtain it later in life from certain drugs and diseases. Men are more likely to be created with it than women.

Your eye doctor can diagnose it with a straightforward test. There's no treatment if you're delivered with it, but special connections and eyeglasses can help many people to inform the difference between certain colors.

- **Uveitis**

This is the name for several diseases that cause inflammation of the uvea (the center layer of the vision which contains the majority of the arteries).

These diseases can destroy eye tissue, and even cause eye loss; symptoms may disappear completely quickly or last for a long period. People with disease fighting capability conditions like AIDS, arthritis rheumatoid, or ulcerative colitis may become more likely to have uveitis. Symptoms can include:

- Blurred vision

- Eye pain

- Eye redness

- Light sensitivity

See your physician if you have these symptoms, plus they don't disappear completely in a few days. They will vary types of treatment for uveitis, with respect to the type you have.

- **Presbyopia**

This happens when you lose the power, despite good way vision, to see close objects. After age 40 roughly, you might have to carry a book or other reading material further from your eyes to make it simpler to read.

Reading glasses, contacts, LASIK, which is laser beam vision surgery, and other methods may be used to restore good reading vision.

- **Floaters**

They are tiny places or specks that float across the field of eyesight; a lot of people notice them in well-lit rooms or outside on a bright day.

Floaters are usually normal; however, they sometimes can be considered a sign of a serious eyesight problem, like retinal detachment. That's when the retina behind your eyes separates from the coating underneath; you could also see light flashes combined with the floaters or a dark shadow run into the advantage of your view.

If you notice an abrupt change in the sort of quantity of areas or flashes you observe or a fresh dark "drape" in your peripheral eyesight, go to your vision doctor at the earliest opportunity.

- **Dry Eyes**

This happens whenever the eyes can't make enough good quality tears. It may feel just like something is in your vision, or like it's burning up, extreme dryness can result in some lack of eyesight.

Some treatments include:

- *Utilizing a humidifier in your house*

- *Special eye drops that work like real tears*

- *Plugs in your rip ducts to reduce drainage*

- *Lipiflow is also another treatment that serves as an*

operation that uses warmth and pressure to take care of dry eyes

- **Testosterone eyelid cream**

Natural supplements with fish oil and omega-3

In case your dry eye problem is chronic, you might have dry eye disease; your doctor could prescribe medicated drops like *cyclosporine (Cequa, Restasis) or lifitegrast (Xiidra)* to stimulate rip production.

- **Excess Tearing**

It has nothing in connection with your emotions; you may be delicate to light, blowing wind, or heat changes. Make an effort to protect your eye by shielding them or putting on sunglasses (go for wraparound structures -- they stop more blowing wind than other styles).

Tearing could also signal a much more severe problem, as *vision contamination or a blocked rip duct*. Your eyesight doctor can treat these conditions.

- **Cataracts**

They are cloudy areas that develop in the vision lens. A healthy zoom lens is clear such as a camera's; light goes by through it to your retina (the trunk of your eyes where images are prepared). When you have a cataract, you can't see as well and could notice glare or a halo around lamps at night.

Cataracts often form slowly; they don't cause symptoms like pain, inflammation, or tearing in the vision. Some stay small and do not affect your view, if indeed they make improvement and impact your eyesight, surgery more often than not works to take it back.

- **Glaucoma**

Your eye is similar to a tire: Some pressure within it is normal and safe, but levels that are too much may damage your optic nerve. *Glaucoma is the name for several diseases that cause this problem.*

A common form is the main open up angle glaucoma; a lot of people who have it don't have early symptoms or pain, so it is important to maintain with your regular vision exams.

It doesn't happen often, but glaucoma can be caused by:

- A personal injury to the vision

- Blocked arteries

- Inflammatory disorders of the vision

- Treatment includes prescription vision drops or surgery.

- **Retinal Disorders**

The retina is a thin coating on the trunk of your eye that comprises cells that gather images and pass them to the human brain; retinal disorders stop this transfer. The retinal disorder varies in different types/conditions listed below:

- Age-related macular degeneration identifies a breakdown of a small part of the retina called the macula.

- Diabetic retinopathy is harm to the arteries in your retina caused by diabetes.

- Retinal detachment happens when the retina

separates from the layer underneath.

It's important to get early diagnosis and also have these conditions treated.

- **Conjunctivitis (Pinkeye)**

In this problem, the tissue that lines the trunk of your eyelids and covering your sclera gets inflamed; it could cause redness, scratching, burning, tearing, release, or a sense that something is in your eyesight.

Folks of all age range can obtain it. Causes include *illness, contact with chemicals and irritants, or allergy symptoms. Wash the hands often to lessen your potential for getting it.*

- **Corneal Diseases**

The cornea is the clear, dome-shaped "window" at the frontend of your eye; it can help to target the light that will come in. Disease, injury, and contact with toxins may cause this damage. Indicators include:

- Red eyes.

- Watery eyes.

- Pain.

- Reduced vision, or a halo effect

The main treatment options include:

- *A fresh eyeglasses or contacts prescription.*

- *Medicated eyes drop.*

- *Surgery*

- **Eyelid Problems**

Your eyelids execute a great deal for you; they protect your eyes, pass on tears over its surface, and limit the quantity of light that can enter.

Pain, itching, tearing, and level of sensitivity to light are normal symptoms of eyelid problems; you could also have blinking spasms or swollen outer sides near your eyelashes.

Treatment could include proper cleaning, medication, or surgery.

- **Vision Changes**

As you grow older, you might find that you can't see as well as you once did; that's normal (you'll probably need eyeglasses or contacts). You might choose to have surgery (LASIK) to improve your vision, if you already have eye glasses; you might need a stronger prescription.

Anytime you have an abrupt loss of eyesight, or everything appears blurry (even if it's short-term), see a medical expert right away.

- **Issues with contact lenses**

They work very well for many individuals; nevertheless, you need to look after them, wash the hands before you touch them, and follow the treatment guideline that was included with your prescription. Also, follow these guidelines:

- Never wet them by putting them in the mouth area. That may make contamination more likely.

- Ensure that your lenses fit properly, so they don't scrape your eyes.

- Use vision drops that say they're safe for contacts.

Never use homemade saline solutions, despite the fact that some lenses are FDA-approved for sleeping in them does not mean you should do it regularly, doing this raises the chance of significant infection.

If you do everything right but still end up having your connections, see your vision doctor. You likely have allergy symptoms, dry eyes, or be better off with eyeglasses. Knowing the actual problem is, you can decide what's right for you.

Chapter 4

Infections of the Eye

If your eyes are itchy and they are starting to change colour of pink, you can call your physician immediately; however, there are fundamental signs that can provide an accurate clues to exactly what is wrong.

Contamination in your eyes can arrive in many various ways. A great deal depends upon which part of your vision gets the problem. For example, you can get symptoms in your;

- Eyelid.

- Cornea (a clear surface that addresses the exterior of your vision).

- Conjunctiva (a thin, moist area that addresses the within of the eyelids and external layer of your eyesight).

Symptoms of the Eye Infection

You might have symptoms in a single or both eyes when you have an infection. Consider this type of trouble:

- Pain or discomfort.

- Itchy eyes.

- A sense that something's on or in your eye.

- Eye hurts if it is bright (light awareness).

- Burning up in your eyes.

- Small, unpleasant lump under your eyelid or at the bottom of your eyelashes.

- Eyelid is sensitive when you touch it.

- Eye won't stop tearing up.

- Discomfort in your eyes.

How your eyes look. You might have changes like:

- Discharge out of 1 or both eyes that's yellow, green,

or clear.

- Red color in the "whites" of your eyes.

- Swollen, red, or crimson eyelids.

- Crusty lashes and lids, especially each day.

You might find you have blurry eyesight. Various other problems you can find are fever, trouble wearing contacts, and swollen lymph nodes near your ear.

Types of Vision Infections

Once you see your physician, you might hear him/her use medical conditions like:

Pinkeye (conjunctivitis): this is the contamination of your conjunctiva and usually provides your eye a red tint. It could be the effect of a bacteria or computer virus, although sometimes you can find it from an allergic attack or irritants. It's common to get pinkeye when you have a cold.

Keratitis: That is the contamination of your cornea. It could be caused by bacteria, infections, or parasites in drinking water; it's a universal problem for individuals who wear contacts.

Stye: It could appear as unpleasant red bumps under your eyelid or at the bottom of your eyelashes. You have them when the essential oil glands in your eyelid or eyelashes get badly infected with bacteria.

Fungal eyes infections: It's uncommon to get attacks from fungi; however, they can be severe if you undertake. Many fungal vision attacks happen after an vision injury, particularly if your vision was scraped with something from an herb, like a stay or a thorn. You can even get one if you wear connections and do not clean them properly.

Uveitis: That is contamination of the center level of your eyesight, called the uvea. It's sometimes associated with an inflammatory disease like arthritis rheumatoid or lupus.

Before deciding on the best treatment for your infection, your physician should take a look at your eye and could also have a tissue or fluid sample. She'll send it to a laboratory, where it gets examined under a microscope or placed into a dish to produce a culture.

Based on the actual lab finds, your physician may recommend medication you take orally, a cream you apply on your eyelid and eyes, or eyes drop (if chlamydia); is because of a personal injury, allergy, irritant, or other health, she may suggest other treatments to cope with those issues. You mustn't wear contacts until your eye infection has solved.

How come there gunk in my eye?

Do you know that you blink 10-20 times one minute? Each time it happens, your eyes get a few milliseconds of safety and quick wetness shower. Blinking also washes away the mucus your eyes make the whole day.

You cannot blink that gunk away when you are asleep, it only gathers in the part of your vision closest to your nasal area (where your lashes meet your eyelid). The correct name for this is ***rheum***; nevertheless, you probably call it rest.

You might place cream-colored mucus once in a while, which is also normal; it forms when an irritant, like fine sand or dirt, gets in your vision. But eye release can sign something you can't blink or wipe away.

Pinkeye: Your eyelid is lined with a see-through membrane called the **conjunctiva**. In addition, it addresses the white part of your eyeball. This coating is filled with tiny arteries you normally can't see. If they get badly infected, the whites of your eye look red or red, hence the name pinkeye. Your physician may possibly also call it conjunctivitis.

It's caused by allergy symptoms or a viral or infection. Vision release is a common sign; babies can obtain it if a rip duct hasn't opened up completely.

Clogged tear duct: You have a rip gland above each eyeball. They make the liquid that gets wiped across your eyesight when you blink. It drains into ducts in the part of your eyes closest to your nasal area. If a rip leave duct is clogged, that liquid has nowhere to visit. The duct can get badly infected and cause release.

Dry vision: Tears are made of four things: **drinking water, natural oils, mucus, and antibodies**. If their balance is off, or if your rip glands stop making tears, your eye gets dry. Whenever your vision doesn't get enough liquid, it tells your anxious system to send some. That sometimes will come in the proper execution of crisis tears, which don't possess the same nourishing balance as regular tears. Crisis tears with too much mucus can result in strings of gunk in or about your eyesight.

<u>*Corneal ulcer*</u>: The cornea addresses your iris, the colored portion of your eyes, as well as your pupil, which allows the light in. It's uncommon, but an ulcer can happen when there's a vision an infection or extreme case of dried out vision; it could create discharge.

Chapter 5

Vision Floaters: Causes, Symptoms, and Treatment

Vision floaters appear as small places that drift through your field of eyesight. They may stick out when you take a look at something shiny, like a white paper or a blue sky. They could annoy you; however, they shouldn't hinder your sight.

When you have a big floater, it can cause a solid hook shadow over your eyesight; but this will happen only using types of light. You can figure out how to live with floaters and ignore them. You might notice them less after a while. Only seldom do they get bad enough to require treatment.

What are the symptoms?

Floaters earn their name by activity in your eyesight. They tend to dart away when you make an effort to concentrate on them.

They come in many different shapes:

- Black or grey dots.

- Squiggly lines.

- Threadlike strands, which may be knobby and almost see-through.

- Cobwebs.

- Rings

Once you have them, they often don't disappear completely. Nevertheless, you usually notice them less as time passes.

What Causes Them?

Most floaters are small flecks of the proteins called **collagen**. They're part of the gel-like substance in the rear of your eyes called the ***vitreous***.

As you age, the protein fibers that define the vitreous shrink right down to little shreds that clump collectively.

The shadows they cast on your retina are floaters; if you see an adobe flash, it's because the vitreous has drawn from the retina. If the floaters are new or significantly transformed or you abruptly start to see flashes, see your vision doctor ASAP.

These changes can occur at any age, but usually occur between 50 and 75. You're much more likely to keep these things if you're nearsighted or experienced cataract surgery.

It's uncommon, but floaters can also derive from:

- Eye disease.

- Eye injury.

- Diabetic retinopathy.

- Crystal-like debris that forms in the vitreous.

- Eye tumors

Serious eye disorders associated with floaters include:

- Detached retina.

- Torn retina.

- Bleeding within your vitreous.

- Swollen vitreous or retina triggered by infections or an autoimmune condition.

- Eye tumors

What might resemble a floater is the *visual aura* that comes with migraine headaches; it could appear to be what it is when you put your vision to a kaleidoscope (it could even move). It's not the same as the floaters and flashbulb type "flashes" that include other eyesight problems. It usually continues a few moments and could involve the eyesight in both eyes. But it completely resolves if you don't have another show.

When to start to see the Doctor

If you have a few eyes floaters that doesn't change as time passes, don't sweat it.

Go directly to the doctor ASAP if you see:

- A sudden upsurge in the number of floaters.

- Flashes of light.

- A loss of aspect vision.

- Changes which come on quickly and worsen over time.

- Floaters after vision surgery or vision trauma.

Eye pain

Choose a general practitioner that has experience with retina problems. If you don't get help immediately, you could lose your view.

How Are Floaters Treated?

Benign ones hardly ever require treatment; if indeed they annoy you, make an effort to have them out of your field of eyesight. Move your eye; this shifts the liquid around.

When you have so many that they stop your eyesight, your eyesight doctor may suggest surgery called a *vitrectomy*; he'll take away the vitreous and replace it with a sodium solution.

It's likely you have complications like:

- Detached retina.

- Torn retina

Cataracts: The chance is low, but if these problems happen, they can permanently harm your vision.

Chapter 6

What are Eye Freckles?

Maybe you've had just a little red color all over your eye because you were a youngster, or maybe you merely discovered you come with a vision freckle throughout a checkup; a freckle in your vision might seem unusual, but they're common and usually safe.

When you have one, your eyesight doctor may choose to watch it as time passes. It's rare; however, they can change into a kind of malignancy called melanoma. So whether they're old or new, it's always smart to have them checked out.

What exactly are they?

Eyes Freckle: There are two types of vision freckles; the first is theoretically known as a *nevus*; they're much like moles on your skin layer. "Nevus" means "mole." A few of these nevi (the plural of nevus) are easy to identify. But others are concealed in the rear of your vision, where nobody but your eyesight doctor will ever see them; they have different titles depending on where they may be:

- *Conjunctival nevus*: On the top of your eye.

- *Iris nevus*: In the colored part of your eye.

- *Choroidal nevus*: Under your retina (in the rear of your eyes)

Nevi can be yellow, dark brown, grey, or a mixture of colours, which are created by special cells called *melanocytes*, which give your skin layer and your eye their color. Those cells are usually disseminated, but if enough of this clump jointly, they form a nevus.

The other kind of eye freckles is called *iris freckles*; they are small flecks in the shaded part of your vision. They're similar to the freckles on your skin layer than moles (they're only on the top of your vision and don't have an effect on its shape); about 50 % of all folks have iris freckles. Some types of nevi form before delivery, while iris freckles will arrive in older adults.

What Causes Eye Freckles?

Doctors don't know why some individuals have them as well as others don't, but a thing or two may impact your chances:

- <u>Competition</u>: Choroidal nevi (in the rear of your eyesight) are a lot more common in white people or people who have lighter skin shades than in dark people.

- <u>Sun Exposure</u>: It's possible that sun harm might increase your likelihood of nevi, and there's evidence that iris freckles are related to being away in the sunlight. A 2017 research found that individuals who spent additional time in sunlight experienced more iris freckles.

Do Eyes Freckles Need Treatment?

Most times, eye freckles are harmless, exactly like most moles and freckles on your skin layer; they're improbable to influence your eyesight or cause any problems. The only reason you may want treatment for an eye freckle is if your physician thinks it could be a melanoma.

See Your Physician

If you've noticed an area or freckle in your eyes, it's most likely not a problem; but it's important to get it tested by a vision doctor (optometrist or an ophthalmologist).

Throughout your appointment, your physician may choose to have a picture of the freckle and perhaps do some imaging scans to check it out more closely. You may want to return every six months or so to ensure the freckle hasn't transformed (like growing bigger). If it still appears the same over time, you often will switch to annual checkups.

Other reasons to see an vision doctor include:

- A freckle in your eyesight that's grown or changed its form or color.

- Eye pain.

- You see blinking lights

Other changes in your vision

To safeguard your eye, wear glasses that stop at least 99% of Ultraviolet rays when you're outdoors. While we don't know for certain, shades might lower the probabilities that a safe nevus will become melanoma. Plus, they definitely decrease your probability of getting cataracts and other serious eye problems.

Chapter 7

Eye Twitch

No one has discovered the cause of this yet, which your physician might call *blepharospasm*. When it happens, your eyelid, usually the top one, blinks, and also you can't make it stop, sometimes it impacts both eyes. The lid moves every couple of seconds for just a few minutes.

Doctors think it could be associated with:

- Fatigue.

- Stress.

- Caffeine

Twitches are painless, harmless, and usually disappear completely independently. If the spasms are strong enough, they can cause your eyelids to shut and then reopen totally. Some individuals have eye spasms the whole day; they might continue for times, days, or even weeks.

It's rare, if a twitch doesn't disappear completely, it might cause you to wink or squint regularly. If you can't keep the eyes open up, it's heading to be hard that you should see.

Sometimes, the twitch can be considered a sign of much more severe conditions, like:

- Blepharitis (inflamed eyelids).
- Dry eyes.
- Light sensitivity.
- Pinkeye

Very rarely, it's an indicator of the brain or nerve disorder, such as:

- Bell's palsy.
- Dystonia.
- Parkinson's disease.
- Tourette's syndrome.

It may also be a side-effect of certain medications; the

most frequent include drugs that treat psychosis and epilepsy.

What are the Types of Twitches?

You will find three frequently occurring ones.

An eyelid twitch is often associated with lifestyle factors, like:

- Fatigue.
- Stress.
- Insomnia.

It can often be caused by the constant usage of alcoholic beverages, cigarettes, or caffeine. Additionally, it may result from the discomfort of the top of your eyes (cornea) or the membranes that collect your eyelids (conjunctiva).

Benign essential blepharospasm usually turns up in the middle to late adulthood and steadily gets worse. Record shows that in 12 month,s not more than 2,000 people suffer from this ailment in America. It isn't a significant condition, but more serious cases can hinder your lifestyle.

Causes include:

- Fatigue.

- Stress.

- Bright light, blowing wind or polluting of the environment.

It begins with non-stop blinking or vision irritation and then gets worse until your eyes become delicate to light and get blurry and also have cosmetic spasms. In serious situations, the spasms may become so extreme that your eyelids stay shut for several hours.

Experts believe it results from a variety of environmental and genetic factors; although the problem is usually arbitrary, it sometimes works in families.

A hemifacial spasm is rare; it entails both muscles around the mouth area as well as your eyelid. Unlike the other two types, it usually impacts only one part of the facial skin. Most often, the reason can be an artery pressing on the facial nerve.

When must I see a medical expert?

Make a scheduled appointment if:

- The twitch is maintained to get more than a week.

- Your eyelid closes completely.

- Spasms involve other face muscles.

- You observe redness, swelling, or release from an eye.

- Your top eyelid drops

If your physician suspects a brain or nerve problem is at fault, she'll look for other common signs; she might send you to a neurologist or other specialist.

How could it be Treated?

Generally, a twitch will recede by itself; ensure you get enough rest and scale back on alcoholic beverages, cigarettes, and caffeine. If dry eye or irritated eye will be the cause, try over-the-counter artificial tears. That may often ease a twitch.

Doctors have still not found an end to benign essential blepharospasm; however, several treatment plans make it less severe. The hottest treatment is *botulinum toxin (Botox, Dysport, Xeomin)*; it is also often used in combination with a *hemifacial spasm*.

A health care provider will inject smaller amounts into your vision muscles to help ease the spasms; the result lasts a couple of months before it gradually wears off, after which you'd have to carry out the treatment over again.

In moderate cases, your physician might suggest medications like:

- Clonazepam (Klonopin).

- Lorazepam (Ativan).

- Trihexyphenidyl hydrochloride (Artane, Trihexane, Tritane)

These usually provide only short-term alleviation.

Alternate treatments include:

- Biofeedback.

- Acupuncture.

- Hypnosis.

- Chiropractic.

- Nutrition therapy.

- Tinted glasses

Scientific tests haven't proven these treatments work.

If other options fail, your physician may suggest surgery; in operation called a *myectomy*, your doctor will remove a few of the muscles and nerves around your eyelid.

Surgery can also relieve the pressure of the artery on your face nerve that triggers a hemifacial spasm.

Chapter 8

Red Spot of the Eye

The red color all over your eye might look frightening, but it's usually no significant offer. There are several tiny arteries between your white of your eyesight and the sclera (the film that addresses it). Sometimes they break.

You will possibly not even remember that you have a red spot (its standard name is sub-conjunctival hemorrhage) until you try looking in a mirror; you won't notice any observable symptoms like eyesight changes, release, or pain. The only soreness you might have is a scratchy sense on the top of your eyes.

What Can Cause Them?

Most happen whenever your blood circulation pressure spikes as a consequence to:

- Strong sneezing.

- Straining.

- Powerful coughing.

- Vomiting

Some red spots derive from a personal injury or illness, like:

- Approximately rubbing your eye.

- Trauma, just like a foreign object stuck in your eye

Contact lenses

- Viral infection.

- Surgery.

    Less common causes include:

- Diabetes.

- High blood circulation pressure.

- Medicines that produce you bleed easily (such as aspirin or bloodstream thinners like Coumadin).

- Bloodstream clotting disorders.

How are they Diagnosed?

Your physician can let you know you have a subconjunctival hemorrhage just from taking a look at your eye.

How Are They Treated?

Most red spots heal independently with no treatment; depending on how big it is, it might take a couple of days or a couple of weeks to disappear completely. If it starts to feel annoying, it's Okay to use artificial tears.

May I Prevent Them?

If you want to rub your vision, get it done gently; if a red place keeps returning, your physician may:

- Ask your questions about your present health insurance and symptoms.

- Do an eye exam.

- Take your blood circulation pressure, execute a routine blood vessels test to be sure you do not have a serious blood loss disorder.

Chapter 9

Diabetes and Eye Problems

As a diabetic patient, the ability to take safety measures in reducing the threat of developing vision problems is essential because blindness is 20 times more prevalent in people who have diabetes. The three major eye problems that individuals with diabetes have to be alert to are *cataracts, glaucoma, and retinopathy*.

To avoid vision problems, you should:

- Control your blood sugar.

- Have your eye checked at least one time a year by an ophthalmologist (eyes specialist).

- Control high blood circulation pressure and lipids.

    Contact your physician if the following happens:

- Dark spots in your vision

- Flashes of light.

Cataracts

A cataract is a clouding or fogging of the zoom lens inside the vision. At these times, light cannot enter the vision and eyesight is impaired.

Symptoms

- Blurred vision
- Glared vision
- Treatment

Treatment - Surgery accompanied by glasses, contacts, or zoom lens implant can help in intense situations like this.

Glaucoma

Glaucoma is an illness of the optic nerve (the "wire" that connects the vision to the mind and transmits light impulses to the mind). If the pressure inside the vision accumulates, it can damage this optic nerve. Often, there are NO symptoms from glaucoma; the following symptoms may occur:

- Loss of eyesight or visual field
- Headaches
- Eye pains (pain)
- Halos around lights
- Blurred vision
- Watering eyes

Treatment

- Special eye drops
- Laser therapy
- Medication
- Surgery

Prevention - Have your eyes doctor display for glaucoma annually.

Retinopathy

Issues with the retina are called *diabetic retinopathy*; this problem is developed consequently when liquid leaks from arteries into the eyesight or abnormal arteries formed in the vision. If retinopathy is not discovered early or is not treated, blindness may appear.

Symptoms

Sometimes there are no symptoms of retinopathy, but two common symptoms are:

- Blurred vision

- Places or lines in your vision

Treatment

- Laser therapy

- Surgery

- Injections into eyes (advanced retinopathy)

Prevention

Have your eyes doctor display the state of your eye on the screen for retinopathy annually.

Women with preexisting diabetes who get pregnant should have a thorough vision exam through the first trimester and close follow-up with an vision doctor during being pregnant, *(This recommendation will not connect with women who develop gestational diabetes, being that they are not in danger for retinopathy.)*

Chapter 10
Glossary of Eye Terms

- *Achromatopsia*: Too little certain receptors in your retinas. Your eyesight won't be razor-sharp, and you will be almost or completely colourblind. It's an inherited condition.

- *Alpha-2 agonists*: Medications used to take care of glaucoma. They help aqueous laughter drain out of your vision and stop your vision from making more of it — the effect: Lower pressure within your eye.

- *Amblyopia*: A disorder also called "lazy eyesight" that begins in child years. Because one or the other vision is not used constantly to give a razor-sharp image, eyesight doesn't develop just how it should. If it isn't treated, one vision will be weaker.

- *Aqueous humor*: The clear, watery liquid in the middle of your lens and cornea.

- *Astigmatism*: Whenever your cornea is shaped similar to a football when compared to a golf ball. It causes blurry eyesight. You are able to correct it with eyeglasses, contacts, or surgery.

- *Beta-blockers*: Medicated vision drops that treat glaucoma. They cause your eyesight to makes less aqueous laughter, and that decreases the pressure within it.

- *Carbonic anhydrase inhibitors*: Medications that treat glaucoma. They cause your eyes to make less aqueous laughter, which decreases pressure.

- *Choroid*: The coating of arteries in the middle of your retina and sclera.

- *Choroiditis*: A kind of uveitis, or irritation of the uvea, the eye's middle level. It causes the coating beneath your retina to be inflamed.

- *Conjunctiva*: A thin level of cells that lines the within of your eyelids and the outer areas of your sclera.

- *Conjunctivitis*: Swelling of your conjunctiva, also known as pinkeye.

- *Cornea*: The clear front side outer coating of your vision; it addresses the iris.

- *Cryotherapy*: Surgery that freezes and destroys abnormal cells.

- *Cyclitis*: A kind of uveitis that inflames the center part of your vision. Additionally, it may have an effect on the muscle that concentrates your zoom lens. Cyclitis will come on instantly and last almost a year.

- *Dilation*: When the vision doctor offers you medicated drops to open up your pupil.

- *Enucleation*: Whenever your vision is surgically removed.

- *Hyperopia*: When it's hard to see items close up, but things farther away are clearer. The usual name because of this is farsightedness.

- *Intraocular*: Of or related to the within of your eyesight.

- *Iris*: The colored membrane around your pupil. It expands and agreements to control the quantity of light that enters your eyes.

- *Iritis*: The most frequent form of uveitis. It impacts the iris, and it is often associated with autoimmune conditions like arthritis rheumatoid. It can arrive suddenly and could last up to eight weeks, despite having treatment.

- *Legal blindness*: Whenever your vision, in both eyes, cannot be corrected or when you have a visible field of 20 levels or less. (Your vision doctor may call this tunnel eyesight.)

- *Low vision*: When you're either legally blind (you have a visible acuity of significantly less than 20/200 or tunnel vision) or have visible acuity between 20/70 and 20/200, regardless of the use of glasses or contacts.

- *Macula*: The central part of your retina, which is

necessary for high res eyesight. When it's healthy, you'll have a clear, sharpened vision.

- *Macular edema*: A swelling of the macula that means it is hard to see. It usually results from damage or disease.

- *Myopia*: If it is difficult to see items in the length while near items have emerged more clearly. Also known as nearsightedness.

- *Nighttime blindness*: When you have trouble viewing in dim or darkened conditions. It could result from too little supplement A. Less often; it's an indicator of retinitis pigmentosa.

- *Nyctalopia*: See night time blindness.

- *Ocular*: Of or related to your vision.

- *Ophthalmologist*: Doctors who focus on the medical and surgical treatment of the eye. They could be either doctor of medication (MD) or doctors of osteopathy (DO). They offer total eye treatment, like eyesight services, eye examinations, medical and medical care, analysis and treatment of disease, and management of problems from other conditions, like diabetes.

- *Ophthalmoscope*: A musical instrument that examines your retina. You can find two types:

- *Immediate*: Examines the guts of your retina.

- *Indirect*: Checks your complete retina.

- *Optic nerve*: It bears light signs from your retina to the human brain, which turns them into images.

- *Optometrist*: A health care provider trained to examine, diagnose, treat, and manage eyesight diseases and disorders. They are able to prescribe eyeglasses and contacts as well as check your eye's inner and external buildings for diseases such as glaucoma, retinal diseases, and cataracts, or common conditions like nearsightedness, farsightedness, astigmatism, and presbyopia. Generally, in most, say they aren't allowed to do laser beam or other eye surgeries.

- *Peripheral vision*: Everything you see from the side of your eye, not your immediate type of vision.

- *Photocoagulation*: A kind of laser beam surgery used to avoid blood loss or repair broken tissue. It's frequently used to take care of retinal conditions like problems from diabetes. In addition, it helps treat vision tumors.

- *Pinkeye*: See conjunctivitis.

- *Presbyopia*: Whenever your eye can't change concentrate to see items up close. It isn't an illness, but an integral part of the eye's natural aging process. It impacts everyone sooner or later in life. It usually turns up around the age group 40 to 45.

- *Pupil*: The circular, dark central starting in your vision. That's where the light will come in.

- *Refraction*: Just how yours eyesight bends light, so a graphic focuses directly on your retina. Also, the task by which your physician determines the optical prescription for contacts or glasses.

- *Refractive error*: Whenever your eyes don't bend light, just how it should. Images are out of concentrate. The most frequent refractive mistakes are astigmatism, farsightedness, and nearsightedness. Your vision doctor can appropriate it with prescription eyeglasses, contacts, or in some instances, laser beam corrective surgery.

- *Retina*: The thin level of nerves that lines the trunk of your vision. It senses light and indicators your optic nerve and brain to produce images.

- *Retinitis pigmentosa*: Some of several retina conditions you can inherit; each makes you lose sight as time passes. Typically a reduction in evening eyesight could be the first indication accompanied by your eyesight tunneling right down to just what the truth is straight forward. Eventually, your central eyesight may decrease.

- *Retinoblastoma*: A malignant tumor that forms on your retina. It frequently happens in children under age 5. It could impact one or both eyes.

- *Sclera*: The outer coating of the eyeball that forms the whites of your eye.

- *Strabismus*: Whenever your eyes are not aligned and can't point in the same path at exactly the same time. The crossed eye is one kind of strabismus.

- *Tunnel eyesight*: Whenever your eyesight is entirely gone, conditions like retinitis pigmentosa and untreated glaucoma can cause tunnel eyesight.

- *Visible acuity*: How you see as measured with a vision chart.

- *Visual field*: Your complete selection of sight, including peripheral vision.

- *Vitrectomy*: With this medical procedure, the vitreous laughter is taken off your eyeball and replaced with a definite sodium solution or temporarily with a gas bubble. It can benefit when marks or bleeding in your vitreous blocks your eyesight.

- *Vitreous humor*: The clear gel-like substance in the heart of your eyeball.

www.ingramcontent.com/pod-product-compliance
Lightning Source LLC
Chambersburg PA
CBHW071123030426
42336CB00013BA/2178